Irritable Bowel Syndrome

IBS Symptoms, Remedies and Prevention

The Alternative Healing Series

Hayden Anderson

This book is dedicated to anyone suffering from Irritable Bowel Syndrome

Copyright Act of 1976, the scanning, uploading and electronic sharing of any part of this book without the explicit written consent or permission of the publisher constitutes unlawful piracy and the theft of intellectual property.

If you would like to use material or content from this book (other than for review purposes), prior written permission must be obtained from the publisher.

You can contact the publishing company at admin@speedypublishing.com. Thank you for not infringing on the author's rights.

Speedy Publishing LLC (c) 2014
40 E. Main St., #1156
Newark, DE 19711
www.speedypublishing.co

Ordering Information:
Quantity sales; Special discounts are available on quantity purchases by corporations, associations, and others. For details, contact the "Special Sales Department" at the address above.

This is a reprint book.

Manufactured in the United States of America

TABLE OF CONTENTS

Publisher's Notes i

Chapter 1: Introduction to Irritable Bowel Syndrome 1

Chapter 2: Irritable Bowel Syndrome Symptoms 3

Chapter 3: Managing Irritable Bowel Syndrome 7

Chapter 4: Stress and Irritable Bowel Syndrome 11

Chapter 5: Irritable Bowel Syndrome and Diet 16

Chapter 6: Understanding Medications to Treat Irritable Bowel Syndrome 26

Chapter 7: Consider Alternative Health Remedies vs. Medications .. 32

Chapter 8: Irritable Bowel Syndrome Prevention 42

Chapter 9: Conclusion - Managing and Preventing Irritable Bowel Syndrome 46

Meet the Author 48

Publisher's Notes

Disclaimer

This publication is intended to provide helpful and informative material. It is not intended to diagnose, treat, cure, or prevent any health problem or condition, nor is intended to replace the advice of a physician. No action should be taken solely on the contents of this book. Always consult your physician or qualified health-care professional on any matters regarding your health and before adopting any suggestions in this book or drawing inferences from it.

The author and publisher specifically disclaim all responsibility for any liability, loss or risk, personal or otherwise, which is incurred as a consequence, directly or indirectly, from the use or application of any contents of this book.

Any and all product names referenced within this book are the trademarks of their respective owners. None of these owners have sponsored, authorized, endorsed, or approved this book.

Always read all information provided by the manufacturers' product labels before using their products. The author and publisher are not responsible for claims made by manufacturers.

Chapter 1: Introduction to Irritable Bowel Syndrome

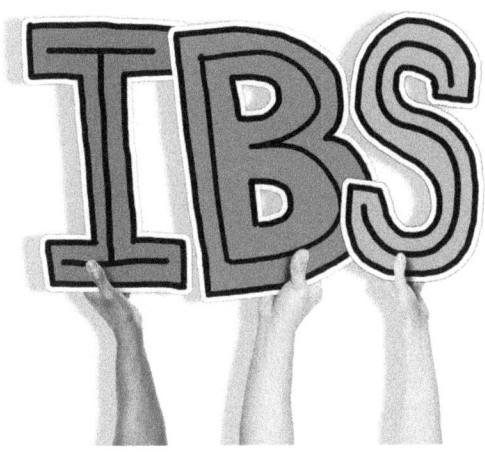

Irritable Bowel Syndrome, also known as IBS, is a condition in which the bowel does not function as it should. If you are one that has been diagnosed with IBS, then there is a real need to find the help to relieve the symptoms you are facing. If you haven't been diagnosed yet, it is time to consider heading to the doctor if you do feel that these are things happening to you.

The problem is that many medications for IBS are not all that safe and can cause unpleasant side effects. Is there a way to safely manage IBS symptoms? How do you go on with your everyday life without having to worry about these symptoms?

What's even more difficult for those that are suffering from IBS, they don't like to talk about their condition. Irritable bowls is not a fun conversation topic.

The good news is that there are some effective means that can help you to relieve the pain and uncomfortableness you face due to IBS. In this book, you will learn how to manage the symptoms of IBS.

Chapter 2: Irritable Bowel Syndrome Symptoms

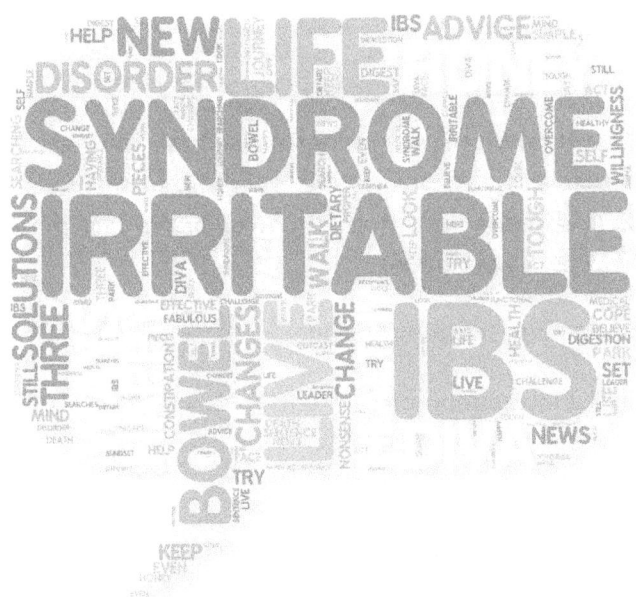

Irritable bowel syndrome is something that no one really wants to talk about, but more people need to hear about.

This condition affects an average of fifty percent of those that visit the gastroenterologist each year. Even if you haven't gone there yet, it is likely that at some point, you might make the trip.

The condition is one that is likely to cause you a great deal of pain and discomfort. For that reason, it is imperative to learn all that you can about what irritable bowel syndrome is as well as how it can be relieved. That's what I aim to do here. But, before you can find relief from irritable bowel syndrome, you must know what it actually is.

What Is It?

IBS, as it is called for short, is also known as spastic colon. In this condition, individuals will experience pain in their abdomen. The pain is due to a disorder of the function of your bowel. In addition to pain, you may also experience changes in normal bowel habits.

IBS Symptoms

There are many symptoms that can be contributed to that of irritated bowel syndrome. Learning about these can help you and your doctor to get a start on what's wrong. In many cases, IBS symptoms may seem like a normal bowel, but in fact there could be additional problems lurking.

The most frequent symptoms include:

- Pain in the lower abdomen
- Bloating
- Pain that is relieved by defecation

If you are suffering from any of these conditions, you may want to talk to your doctor, especially if they are recurring.

The symptoms that you may experience may feel like diarrhea or even constipation. In some individuals it moves from one extreme to the next. A change in the stool is often a symptom of IBS.

It is also believed that those that have other conditions are more likely to experience IBS. Those conditions include chronic fatigue syndrome, stress, chronic pelvic pain and fibromyalgia.

Some doctors have found that there is a link between irritable bowel syndrome and mental conditions. They link IBS to having both neurological and psychological components.

In addition to this, conditions can make it worse. For example, menstruation usually makes IBS worse or makes the symptoms more pronounced.

What To Do First

If you believe that you are suffering from Irritable Bowel Syndrome, it is imperative that you work on getting the relief you need. The first step is to be diagnosed by your doctor.

Most doctors will be able to provide you with the necessary testing and evaluation. Your doctor will want to track your bowel movements over a period of time as well as monitor your other conditions during the monitoring.

There are several things that they will look at.

1. Are you relieved from the pain after defecation?
2. When you feel this way, is there a change in the frequency of your stool?
3. When you are experiencing this pain, is there a change in the form or the way that your stool looks?

Then, they will gauge the differences and answers found with what is considered to be normal against what is not.

- If you have more than three bowel movements per day or you have less than three movements per week, that is considered abnormal.
- If you have hard or lumpy stool or you have a very loose and watery stool that is considered abnormal.
- If you are straining, or you have an urgent need to go or you feel like you can not completely finish, this too is abnormal.
- If there is any sign of mucus, this is abnormal.
- In addition, the feeling of pain in the abdomen or the feeling of being bloated is considered abnormal.

Through the screening process your doctor is likely to do a blood work up on you as part of the process of diagnosing you.

Finally, your doctor will do a thorough examine of you. The exam will look at your physical conditions to rule out any other possible findings that may suggest something besides irritable bowel syndrome is to blame for your pain.

When It's Not IBS

Your doctor may actually find that you have symptoms that don't present within irritable bowel syndrome. These symptoms can include blood within the stool, weight loss, fevers, diarrhea that gets you up at night or pain that gets you up at night. These problems indicate that perhaps something else is wrong rather than IBS.

Where The Truth Lies

Unfortunately, there is no known cause for irritable bowel syndrome. Many that experience it do not know of anyone in their family that has had it. That could be because it just wasn't something that was discussed or that IBS is not hereditary.

There are things that are known about IBS, though, that can help you to find the real solution to your pain and discomfort. We do know a great deal about how IBS affects us and what we can do to help to stop it.

Chapter 3: Managing Irritable Bowel Syndrome

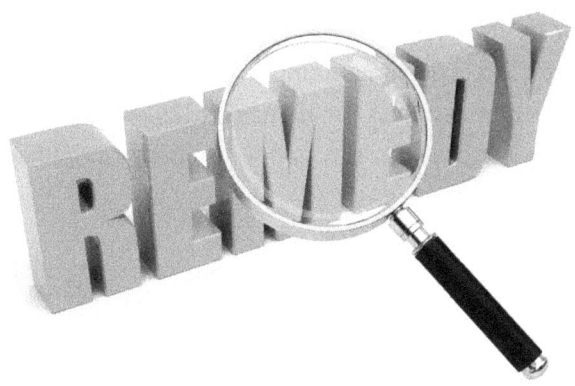

Irritable bowel syndrome is not something that has a one-hundred percent cure rate. In most cases, you and your doctor will work at determining how best to tackle and handle the symptoms. Without the cause being known, there is little that can be done to remove the pain and discomfort forever once and for all.

One thing that should be noted is that irritable bowel syndrome is not a progressive condition. It is also not life threatening to those that suffer from it. There is no reason to believe that you can't get help and will have to suffer with IBS either.

There is a lot that can be done to help improve the quality of your life by handling the symptoms that you face.

How To Manage IBS

There is a lot to think about when it comes to managing IBS. There are medications, home remedy solutions and other things that you will need to do to help stop the pain and suffering that you are experiencing.

In most cases, you can get some relief by implementing just one of the types of treatments available to you. But, most that suffer from IBS will want to consider doing more than just adding one treatment to their regimen for managing IBS. With a constant eye on several key factors, you can find a number of benefits in health related costs.

Treatments To Be Considered

There are several types of treatments that can be used in the relief of irritable bowel syndrome. In later chapters, we will go into full details about each of these so that you can adapt them into your lifestyle and find the relief that you need.

- Stress relief
- Your diet
- Prevention of the condition
- Self care measures
- Coping with the condition
- Medications prescribed
- Alternative medications available
- Complementary treatments

Each of these avenues is something that you should carefully consider if you are to overcome what IBS can do to you. In addition to this, the severity of your condition should be taken into considerations.

Those that suffer from more extreme cases are going to need more help than those that do not. Your treatment should be based on just how extreme your condition is. In effect, the treatment for a mild case of IBS is not going to be enough for those with severe symptoms. Likewise, the treatment for severe IBS is not going to be beneficial to those that are suffering from a mild condition.

What's What?

Your doctor will work with you in diagnosing and then determining what level of severity your IBS is. For each person, this will mean meeting with and following up on your doctor's diagnosis.

But, you can learn more about your condition by monitoring the levels of your condition on your own. Once you know to what degree you are suffering, there is a simple set of tools available to you to use.

If you have mild IBS, your goal will be to work through management of stress factors and to make changes to the foods that you eat and to your overall lifestyle.

For those that are suffering from more moderate conditions of IBS, there is a need to make the changes noted above for mild conditions as well as to take fiber supplementation, anticholinergic medications (or those similar to them) and possibly over the counter relief.

If you do have a severe form of IBS, you'll need to follow both the mild and moderate conditions, but in addition, you will need to talk to your doctor about further medications. These can include tricyclic or SSRI antidepressants or other types of medication.

How Do You Know?

The biggest question that most individuals with IBS ask themselves is a simple, how do I know what to do? The best answer that can be given is to meet with and talk to your family doctor first. If you don't find answers there, more on to working with a specialist in the field.

Through a series of testing, your doctors will help you to fully understand your condition including the severity of your symptoms. Once that is complete, they will help you to make the right lifestyle changes and, in most cases, you will also be prescribed medications to manage it.

The recommendations of a specialist in the field are by far the very best way to go. He or she will aid you in providing the right treatment for your specific condition, not just the symptoms that are most common with irritable bowel syndrome.

But, it makes sense to keep yourself completely updated and educated on what is happening in the world of IBS.

In the next chapters of this book, you will learn various methods to managing your IBS condition. In most cases, you will want to consider making the necessary changes to your lifestyle that will make a significant difference to your IBS symptom severity as well as its frequency. Dedicate your time to improving your lifestyle and diet, and you will most likely find relief.

As for medications, make sure that you discuss with your doctor the types of medications that can help in your specific situation as not all of them are right for everyone.

Chapter 4: Stress and Irritable Bowel Syndrome

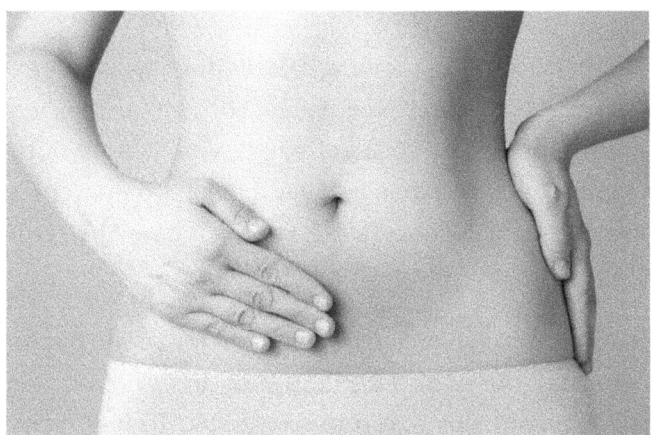

One of the first things that you and your doctor will talk about in regards to your IBS is stress. Stress if a factor that can do damage to many aspects of your health including irritable bowel syndrome.

First and foremost, don't make the mistake of thinking that stress in and of itself can cause IBS. This is not the case. Stress is generally brought into our lives by a troubled lifestyle. The more stress you have, the less likely your body will be at fighting off illness and symptoms.

Remember that we don't know what actually causes IBS. In effect, all we can do is to treat the symptoms that can come from it. But, we do know what makes it worse and stress is one of those factors.

Why Stress Hurts

The facts on why stress hurts your IBS are clear. For a healthy person in an ideal situation, stress is controlled by the body. Your body has a pain inhibition system that turns on when it is struggling with pain to help you to cope with it.

But, what has been found in patients with IBS is that this hypersensitivity doesn't go away. Your body doesn't turn on the right pain inhibition system and you feel the muscles of your gut hurting.

For example, it has been a long and stressful day, you are looking forward to a good meal and sleep. If you are experiencing prolonged or repeated episodes of stress, you'll find it not so easy to relax. Instead, you go home and eat a meal. No matter if you eat during your stressful event or after, your will have that awful ache in your abdomen that comes with IBS.

This would be a normal feeling of being full for some, but for those with IBS it hurts. Your body doesn't turn off the pain function that a healthy body would which in turn allows you to feel more of the pain associated with eating during or after stress.

It Doesn't Have To Be Food

Don't think that the only reason that the IBS pain is brought on only from food. In fact, there have been studies done to provide this. For example, your body experiences a normal emotional response to a situation. In people, the experience of emotional reactions is not something that is strictly emotional. Your body reacts in many ways.

If you are afraid, nervous or sad, your body reacts physically as well as emotionally. Your heart starts to race. Your hands are sweaty. You feel the need to use the restroom. You may even get a nervous, anxious feeling in the pit of your stomach.

In IBS patients, those symptoms intensify for the stomach pain. We know that the body reacts to emotional feelings and stressful situations bring out pronounced pain in the stomach's walls. Your gut may hurt to the point where it is quite troublesome.

In these examples, you can see that no matter what the stressful situation is to your body, it plays a role in making your symptoms far from ordinary. In effect, your IBS is made worse by these conditions.

For that reason, the avoidance of stressful situations can be quite helpful at reducing the number of painful episodes that you go through.

The question is, then, how can you avoid all of the stressful events in your life?

What you need to remember here is that it is not just a matter of avoiding stressful events to stop IBS, but to lower the body's reactions to them. To make it less severe of a reaction, you need to avoid stress and you need to do things that help to relieve stress that you are already facing.

When you do those two things, you can find relief from some of your worst IBS situations. The question is now, how can you do this.

Removing Stress

There is no doubt that removing stress from your lifestyle is going to be challenging. And, there is no doubt that each of us will face stressful situations no matter what we do to avoid them. But, it isn't all about avoiding those situations.

In many ways, doing things that will relieve your stress will help your IBS to find less of a reason to act up. You see, it is the added stress in your body that makes IBS react, not necessarily just one or two stressful situations. Although, in an extreme case, that is all it will likely take to have a reaction.

Here are some of the best ways for you to work on relieving stress in your life.

Avoidance: Of course, the best thing to do is to remove yourself from situations that are always stressful to you. If your job is causing you to lose sleep at night or causing constant worry, then this will lead to IBS reactions. Since your job is an ongoing thing, it builds up and causes your IBS to act up. In situations like this, the only way to find relief from constant stress is to remove it if possible.

Exercise: Believe it or not, your body can relax and find benefit in exercise. This is a great way for you to reduce the stress in your body. Try to get in a walk each day after dinner. Or, sign up for a membership at the local gym and do some laps in the pool. Getting in physical activity does much more than just help you to stay fit. It also helps to stimulate the brain which in turn helps your body reduce stress.

Meditation: For some, mediation is a great way to find relief from stress. Focusing on the good things instead of always worrying about the bad things is the perfect way to find relief from stressful events. If you don't feel that mediation is right for you, try yoga. This will combine both meditation and exercise to provide ideal stress relief to your body and to your mind.

Do Something Fun: Even when things are really looking bad, your mind needs to focus on other things that are beneficial. If you can get out with your friends for a night and have some fun, that will help to take some of the stress away. Everyone needs to find things to do that takes their mind off of the stress they are under.

Get Enough Sleep: A very important part of fighting stress is taking care of your body's physical needs. Sleep is not an option but a requirement for good health. By getting in enough sleep so that you feel rested when you wake up will help your body to cope with stress as it goes throughout your day.

Reducing stress is a great way to help you to avoid irritable bowel syndrome. There is little doubt that having the right physical and emotional outlets will allow you to feel better and get through the day without having the symptoms of IBS.

Use these methods to help you to reduce your stress load. Keep in mind that there are plenty of other ways that you can reduce stress. You just need to maintain a healthy living environment. If you do not take the time to reduce and avoid stress in your daily life, IBS will be a constant factor.

Remember that stress is not the only thing that you need to think about. Pair stress reduction or removal with other necessary considerations and you will quickly see the rewards.

Chapter 5: Irritable Bowel Syndrome and Diet

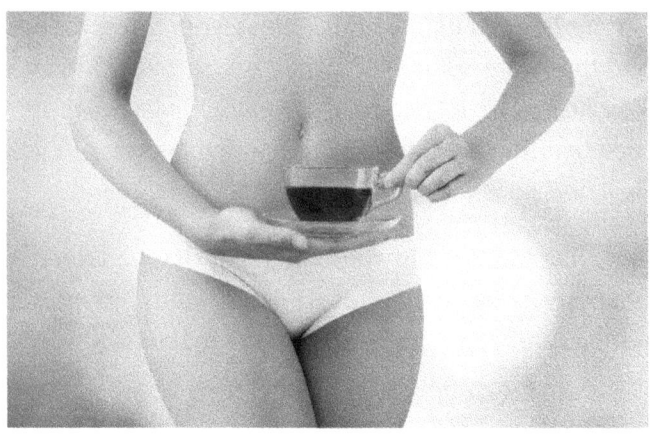

Like stress, your diet does not bring on IBS. Although many people think that they have caused this condition by eating less than healthy foods, that is not the case. Yet, it is well known that foods can contribute to making irritable bowel syndrome worse.

Your body may react to some foods in a more intense way with IBS than others would react to that food. In addition, the body experiences increased levels of intestinal muscle reaction and sensitivity with IBS than otherwise. Just the fact that you are eating can make the symptoms of IBS show themselves. It may not even be a specific food that is causing it, but a general overreaction to food.

The Problems with Foods

The first thing to work on is the simple fact that you can control what you eat. In that, you can have some control over how your body reacts with IBS symptoms. Some of the foods that we know are problematic for those with IBS include foods like fried foods, alcohol, caffeine and foods that are high in fat. In addition to this, when too much food is consumed at one sitting, problems can also arise.

Diarrhea and cramping in your abdomen can be caused by some specific types of sugars that are unable to be fully digested by the bowel. These include sorbitol which is a sweetener in dietetic foods, gum sugars, candy sugars, and fructose. The consumption of these sugars will lead to the inability of the bowel to absorb them correctly and will lead to diarrhea.

The gas symptoms of IBS can be brought on by some foods as well. For example, beans, legumes, cauliflower, lentils, Brussels sprouts, onions, bagels, cabbage and broccoli all can bring on more intense gas like symptoms of IBS. Eating these types of foods can bring on the symptoms of IBS including bloating and increased gas.

With these foods being behind the onset of symptoms of IBS, it is important for you to consider how they affect you. It is essential for you to understand that foods affect each person in a different way. What affects you and causes intense symptoms of IBS may not have the same effect on another person with IBS symptoms. For that reason, it is critical that you find out how foods affect you.

Tracking Your Diet

One of the best first steps for you to do in managing IBS is to track your diet. Although you may think you know what you're eating, you may not realize the correlation between your diet and your IBS symptoms. The goal is to learn what worsens your symptoms.

You should track your diet for two to three weeks solidly. That means writing down everything that is eaten for a full two weeks at least. You'll also need to monitor what you felt like before and after those meals as well as what IBS symptoms you experienced.

A tracking chart will aid you in tracking the foods that you eat each day and the way that you feel before and after each meal. By doing this, you will be able to see that certain foods seem to bring on your IBS symptoms more so than others.

Elimination Diets

As you work through monitoring your food intake, you are likely to find common areas where there is a food you are consuming that seems to be causing additional or worsened IBS symptoms. When that type of food is found, and there is no doubt that when you eat it you feel bad, remove it from your diet.

But, if you do this because you think that the food is causing the problem when in fact it may not be, there is no reason to remove the food from your diet. The hard part is telling the difference.

Since your diet is such a large factor for most in the type of IBS lifestyle they will lead, it does pay to use a chart to help you to track your intake and the symptoms you experience after eating that food. Remember, there is also concern about over eliminating foods in your diet.

The first concern is that the individual is losing quality of life by not eating all of the foods that he or she would like to eat. If this is done without a positive benefit on your lifestyle such as reduced IBS symptoms, then there is no benefit to you and no reason to be so limiting.

Elimination diets can be a problem in and of themselves as well. For many individuals that remove too many of the necessary nutrients that they need from their diet there are the risk of health concerns.

Some individuals can suffer from anemia, osteoporosis and even can suffer vitamin and mineral deficiencies to a great extent.

In addition to this, diets that actually recommend removing entire food groups should be avoided. This includes diets that remove all fats, all proteins or all carbohydrates from your diet, or most of them. This is just not healthy in any type of diet.

If you will be using an elimination diet to help you to find the foods that are not good for your IBS situation, you should be doing so with the help of your doctor or dietician.

If there is some reason for you or your doctor to believe that food is behind your condition to an extreme level, he or she will do testing such as allergy testing, upper intestinal endoscope, and lactose breathing testing.

There are some conditions in which your body will have intolerance for the food which is likely to cause you to feel IBS symptoms more readily. Through testing your doctor will determine if you are suffering from one of these conditions as well.

Some that are common with IBS include:

- GERD, or Gastro esophageal reflux disease which is chronic reflux of gases into the esophagus.
- Celiac Disease which is called a gluten enteropathy is a condition of which there is a reaction between gluten and the muscle lining of the intestine.
- Lactose intolerance is a condition in which the ability to digest milk is not possible.
- Food allergies which is a response from your immune system to the food by which you are eating.
- Eosinophilic Gastroenteritis is a rare condition in which there is a reaction to food that causes white blood cells to enter the GI tract and causes illness.

Through testing, your doctor with your help will determine if you have any of these conditions which can worsen the symptoms you are facing with irritable bowel syndrome symptoms.

Monitoring Intake

In addition to the types of foods that you consume, also take note of just how much you have eaten. Learning what portion sizes are recommended is also essential to the patient with IBS.

With IBS, symptoms can be brought on or made worse by the fact that you are consuming too much food at one sitting. Although most Americans don't realize it, most of the foods we eat are far too much for one sitting. Not only does this contribute to being overweight but it also causes problems with digestion.

Remember the example of eating a full meal and feeling the symptoms of IBS coming on just from eating? That is due to the over sensitivity of your body due to IBS. Because your body doesn't stop the pain reaction as it should, you can experience extreme pain from just overeating.

The question that many have to face then; is what is the right amount of a food they plan to eat?

One way to learn this is to use packaging labels to help you. Learn how much food is considered to be one portion. Food labels make this easy by allowing you to divide the serving size amount the noted servings. For example, if the package says that there are four servings in that package, divide the finished product in four before serving to yourself or to others.

Common Portion Sizes

Here are some of the portions you may want to take control of when it comes to monitoring your IBS symptoms. This is a great way to estimate how much you should eat.

Fruit: One cup, one cup of fruit looks like the size of a baseball.

Salad: One cup, one cup of salad looks like the size of a baseball.

Bread: A slice of bread is one serving.

Pasta, rice or potatoes: One ½ cup is a serving. This looks like the size of half of a baseball.

Pancakes: One pancake is a serving and looks like the size of a compact disc.

Meats: Fish, poultry, beef, pork or other meats, three ounces is one serving and is the size of a deck of playing cards.

Grilled or baked fish: three ounces is a serving and will look like the size of a check that fits into a checkbook.

Ice cream: One ½ of a cup is a serving, and is the size of ½ a baseball.

Milk: One cup is a serving and is the size of your fist

Cheese: 1 ½ ounces is a serving. It looks like four dice stacked.

Oils used for cooking or greens: serving is one teaspoon, which is the size of the tip of your thumb.

Now, look at these sizes. How often do you eat the right portion of meat or pasta? How often do you overeat on these foods and find yourself facing the symptoms of irritable bowel syndrome?

That's Not Enough!

Many people will react to this portion control measure with the fear that there is no way that the amount of food within a portion is enough to fill them.

There are some things that contribute to how much food you should eat. Yes, for some, there is a need to eat more. Here are some factors that play a role in how much you need to eat.

- Men need to eat more than women due to size and muscle mass.
- Those that get more physical activity than thirty minutes per day of activity need to increase these amounts somewhat to compensate.
- Children and teens need to consume more as they are growing.
- Elderly individuals may need additional calories depending on what they are doing physically during the day.

How can you know how much is the right amount of food for you? The best way to monitor the food intake you should be consuming is simple. Ask your family doctor how many calories you should be consuming per day. The physically active male should consume about twenty-two hundred per day. The physically active female should consume about eighteen hundred calories per day.

Tips For Eating Less

Worried that you'll not be able to control the amount that you eat? Here are some great tips for making sure that every bite counts but doesn't hurt in the process. Here are some tricks:

1. Pay attention to how much you are eating. Don't sit down with a large plate of food.
2. Use eight inch plates instead of larger plates as these smaller plates won't allow you to eat so much in one helping. They trick the mind.
3. Eat slowly. Take the time to taste each bite of food you eat.
4. Instead of bringing all of the food to the table, leave all food dishes at the counter and come to the table with just a plate of food. You won't be tempted to eat what's left over.
5. Pay attention to how frequently you are eating. Are you consuming more than you realize with bites of snacks here or there?

These tips can help you to reduce the amount of food you are eating. Paying attention to this, in turn, helps you to reduce the amount of and the intensity of the symptoms of IBS that you face.

Over Limiting Yourself

Did you know that you can do damage to your health if you overtly limit yourself when it comes to IBS dietary restrictions? There is no need to go to such lengths as to be on very specific diets of food. When you limit yourself to such a degree, you only set yourself up to actually fail. Diets or plans that are too strict and limiting to you are much harder to follow and stay on.

In addition, some of these diets require the replacement of full food groups. That in itself is not acceptable because it limits the nutrition that you are getting as well.

Instead of these things, you'll want to take into consideration which foods bring on IBS symptom severity and limit or remove those from your diet. Otherwise, a well balanced diet is the other ingredient to a healthy lifestyle and shouldn't be restricted in the process.

Even still, there are many suggestions of very strict diets for IBS patients. Unless your doctor recommends one of these for your severe irritable bowel syndrome conditions, it is not advisable to use them.

The Best IBS Diet Suggestions For All

It all comes down to understanding what the best possible foods for you to eat are. While each person will experience feedback from their body, most can benefit from these specific changes:

- Drink at least sixty-four ounces of water per day.
- Consume the right amount of fiber.
- Reduce the amount of highly fatty foods and fried foods in your

diet.
- Instead of three large meals, eat six smaller ones and don't snack in between.
- Remove foods with fructose and sorbitol from your diet or limit them strictly.
- Reduce the amount of alcohol and caffeine in the diet to as low as possible.

Doing these things is likely to help improving your diet and therefore improve your overall health including the reduction in IBS symptoms.

Considering Fiber

When it comes to IBS, many individuals need to carefully manage their fiber intake. Too much fiber leads to diarrhea where as not enough can cause constipation. What do you need?

The best thing to start with is to consume a variety of different types of fiber. You should consume fiber from fruits, whole grains and from vegetables. The best way to actually get your fiber and benefit from its overall ability is through these natural resources.

Your body needs fiber for several reasons. For example, the gas that is produced by fiber is necessary to stimulate your colon muscles as well as to help soften your stool.

But, for some individuals that have IBS, this does cause a number of problems in the process. Adding too much fiber is usually the reasoning behind the discomfort that you face. For that reason, you should start to consume additional fiber from your regular diet slowly, monitoring how much you are getting in any one day.

The best ways to get these specific fiber additives is to consume foods that contain them including citrus foods, flaxseeds and legumes.

Conclusion

The end result is that the foods you eat, both good and bad, affect the way that your body reacts. By finding out what foods cause you to suffer and removing or limiting them, you can clearly see benefits in the long term when it comes to your overall health. By eating a well balanced diet and restricting foods that trigger your IBS symptoms, you can improve how often and how severe those symptoms can be.

Chapter 6: Understanding Medications to Treat Irritable Bowel Syndrome

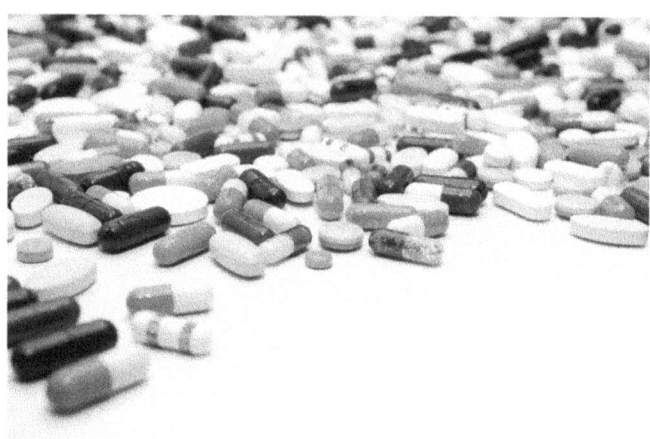

Irritable bowel syndrome is a condition that has several medicinal choices for relief. In most cases, these medications are not given to everyone, but to those with a moderate to extreme level of IBS symptom severity. In other words, they may not be the right choice for you.

These medications come in several forms and you may have heard a lot about them when you visit your doctor to become diagnosed with IBS in the first place.

If your doctor did not mention them, or you are not sure if they are right for you, talk with your doctor. Your individual situation may warrant a different medication or just lifestyle changes to manage your symptoms.

It can't be said enough that the biggest benefit to managing IBS symptoms comes not from medication treatments, but rather from the use of lifestyle and dietary changes in your everyday life. Making changes to your stress levels help as well.

If these changes are not enough, then you may be eligible for medication. For those individuals, let's break down the options that are available to them.

The First Line

The first line of medications is over the counter. In many cases, your IBS symptoms may be mild and there is no need for prescription treatment. Some of the medications and treatments that may be helpful to you include these:

- **Fiber supplements.** As we mentioned earlier, fiber is a critical part of maintaining health. In the case of IBS, the right amount of fiber is required to provide the individuals with necessary help in relieving constipation. Fiber supplements may be the best route to this. There are two types. Psyllium which is like the brand name Metamucil and methylcellulose which is like the brand name of Citrucel.

- **Anti-Diarrhea Medications.** These are medications for the opposite effect. They will work to control diarrhea. You can purchase loperamide such as the brand name Imodium to help with the diarrhea that your IBS symptoms may produce.

Prescription Medications

As we mentioned, there are a few options when it comes to providing relief for IBS symptoms in the way of prescription medications.

There are a few that are used in the same as anti-diarrhea medications and fiber is used.

- **Anticholinergic Medications.** These medications can help with problems with your nervous system. For some individuals with IBS, there is a need for medication that can help regulate the activities of the nervous system. These are called anticholinergics. They provide relief from uncomfortable and even painfully spasms of the bowel.

- **Antidepressant Medications.** For some individuals, there is a need for this medication because of the depression and pain that they are experiencing. If this is found to be the case, your doctor may give you a tricyclic antidepressant or a serotonin reuptake inhibitor which is also called an SSRI. These help with the depression symptoms but they also help with controlling the intestines through the neurons within your brain. This includes tricycle antidepressants for diarrhea and abdominal pain. Others, such as Prozac and Sarafem and Paxil are used to help with depression as well as pain and constipation.

In addition to working with your doctor about your IBS condition, you may also be benefited by working with a counselor as well. This is a common situation for those that can't find help from the antidepressant medications that they are taking. In some cases, relief can be found for these needs through counseling.

Medications Designed for IBS

There are a number of medications that can be helpful to those that are facing IBS. These medications may or may not be right for you. Your doctor will work with you to determine which ones are the best possible tools to help relieving your severe IBS symptoms.

There are two drugs that are currently being used to treat IBS. They are Alosetron, with brand name Lotronex and Tegaserod which is branded as Zelnorm.

Alosetron

This medication is one that is quite controversial in its use. In November of 2000, the Food and Drug Administration removed it from the market. Before then, there were at least 197 individuals that had severe side effects due to taking this medication and there were four deaths that were attributed to it as well. It was only on the market for a mere nine months time.

But the FDA decided to once again allow Alosetron on the market with some restrictions in place in June of 2002. This medication is to be used as a nerve receptor antagonist. Its goal is to relax the colon enough and slow the movement of waste through the lower bowel, thereby helping to relieve many of the symptoms of IBS.

Today, it is only strictly prescribed to female patients. Only women are able to get this medication as men are not approved for it. In addition, only doctors that have received specialized training with the drug's use can prescribe it. It is only to be used in severe cases in which the individual has diarrhea predominant IBS. Patients should be sure that any other method of treatment of their IBS symptoms was not helpful.

If your doctor prescribes this medication to you, it is essential to talk to him about the possible side effects and to monitor your condition closely to insure that you are not suffering from anything that could be life threatening or drastic.

Tegaserod

The second type of medication that is used to treat IBS is that of tegaserod. It is well known for its commercial marketing as the brand name Zelnorm. This medication has been shown to be effective in helping with IBS in several ways. Those that have constipation IBS will find this to be beneficial.

The medication works by imitating the action of the neurotransmitter serotonin. This helps to get the nerves and the muscles in the intestines on the same track and therefore relieves constipation.

There are some studies that have shown that tegaserod is capable of providing severe side effects in some individuals. If your doctor prescribes this medication for you, you should monitor your condition for any side effects. Should be find anything to be severe, it is essential that you talk with your doctor as soon as possible to insure that the medication was the right choice for you.

If you do begin to take any of these medications for your IBS treatment, it should be done only after you have successfully implemented lifestyle changes, dietary changes as wells as stress management.

In addition to this, you should have seen a specialist in the field and he or she should do the prescribing of this medication. Because the medications are potentially dangerous, it is import for you to be properly placed on them.

Other Options

There are some additional medications in the works for IBS suffers. A drug that is similar to that of Alosetron is in clinical trials currently.

In addition, the medication Kappa-opioid Agonish (Fedotozine) is in studies and may be available in a few years. This medication is one that is a synthetic narcotic which will help to reduce the pain in the intestines. It is similar to an opiate.

Another medication called Alpha-2 Adrenergic Agents is in the works as well. This medication should be available in a few years if it is approved by the FDA. It works by making bowel function normal as well as relieving the pain associated with IBS.

Is medication for you? There are still other options available to you to help you to fight IBS. Read on.

Chapter 7: Consider Alternative Health Remedies vs. Medications

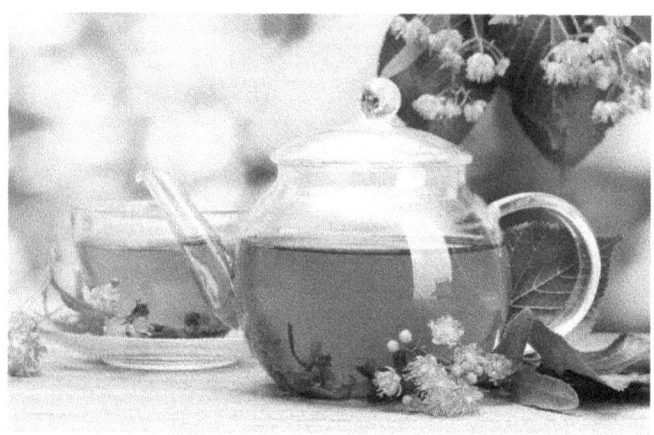

We've talked a lot about the medications and the lifestyle changes that you need to make in order to manage irritable bowel syndrome. It goes without saying that it can be one of the most challenging conditions to deal with because there are so many concerns about medications.

There are some excellent alternative treatments and herbal remedies that have shown some help with handling the symptoms of IBS.

As with all alternative treatments, there is no guarantee that these will work for you. Some treatments seem to help others more so than others. Yet, when it comes to finding relief from IBS, it goes without saying that any type of treatment that has the potential of helping should be fully explored.

In this chapter, we'll dive into some of those alternative treatment options. In many cases, you'll be able to pair them along side your other treatments for added benefit from IBS.

Why Use Alternative Treatments?

There are many different alternative treatments for all conditions out there. From the common cold to fighting cancer, and yes, IBS too, there is an alternative treatment that can be helpful to you. Why should you consider using alternative treatments, then?

There are many reasons and the largest reason that others find it important to use alternative treatments is simple. Most alternative treatments, especially herbal remedies and the like don't have the harsh side effects that chemical medications do.

In the wake of many of the different problems with IBS medications, more and more individuals are looking for alternative methods of managing their IBS other than through prescriptions.

Complementary Therapies

You will want to consider complementary therapies when looking for alternatives to the medications for IBS. As the word implies, complementary treatments can safely be taken with other medications or other changes in your lifestyle.

In many cases, they are taken in addition to medications which make the end result just that much better for the IBS sufferer.

Some of the complimentary therapies that you should consider implementing into your daily lifestyle to fight IBS include:

- Herbal and dietary products
- Somatic therapies such as acupuncture
- Breathing and movement therapies
- Mind body therapies

When used in virtually any health consideration, there can be benefits from these therapies to the patient. In many cases, there are no adverse side effects or unbelievably difficult procedures to go through.

Complementary treatments allow you to be treated as a whole person rather than treating only the symptoms that you are experiencing. There are many people that do not agree with what their doctors say or just don't like the approach that is being taken. In many ways, using complimentary treatments allows you to stay in control of your own treatment.

Now, let's break down the various types of complimentary therapies that you can consider for treatment of IBS. Remember, using any or all of these methods can improve your overall health and well being.

Herbal Therapy

Herbal therapy is a therapy that uses naturally found plants and plant products to aid in making someone feel well. In many cases, the herbal remedies that you will find have been used for thousands of years by ancient Chinese civilizations. Some of them have worked, some of them have not.

The herbal therapies that are designed for IBS, there are generally more than one set of ingredients or therapies. This is because of how the therapies are used. Instead of looking at the disease and its progress, ancient remedies instead look at the pattern of symptoms that you are facing and address this.

Of course, it is important to realize that most of the herbal treatments available today have been modified over time. Not only because of the ingredients available but also how the condition has changed over that period of time as well.

The most commonly used herbs for irritable bowel syndrome include:

- Licorice
- Cardamom
- Rhubarb
- Barley
- Tangerine peel
- Barley

When you purchase them, it is likely that they will contain five or more herbs in one form. When purchasing these, it is of the utmost importance to pay attention to who you are purchasing them from and the quality of the product.

Without the highest quality and purest forms of these herbal treatments, it is unlikely that you will see the benefits that are available through the use of them otherwise. Stay away from products that have synthetic ingredients.

If you don't believe that they work, then you have nothing to lose in trying them. In fact, there have been studies done that actually have shown improvement in IBS patients that received a dosage of herbal products daily over time. Most of them came back to be reassessed with improved symptoms.

Here are some additional herbal supplements that you can take that have shown to provide some improvement for IBS in the patient.

Ginger

Ginger is a common food to be consumed with regard to relieving IBS problems. The use of ginger can be done in several ways. For those with IBS, a treatment can be to use ginger extract. A few drops of this consumed daily can help by providing anti-inflammatory conditions as well as improving the quality of the lining of your gastric system and helping the intestines to do their job.

Peppermint Oil

A common treatment for gastrointestinal conditions is that of peppermint oil. You should be careful when consuming large amounts of peppermint oil as it can cause some individuals to have heartburn. Otherwise it can be beneficial to those suffering from IBS.

When used to treat IBS, peppermint oil is helpful in several ways. It can help to decrease the amount of muscle spasm that your GI tract undergoes. In addition, it can help with the other common symptoms of IBS such as relieving bloating and pain in the abdomen.

Add a few drops of peppermint oil to your drink and you'll have a nice tasting treatment for your IBS symptoms that might be lurking in your day.

Artichoke Leaf Extract

Throughout Europe, artichoke leaf extract has been useful in treating IBS. It has shown some improvements in the secretion of bile by the sufferer. There hasn't been a lot of study about this treatment as of yet, though.

Others

There are other herbal products that you can take to help you with constipation. Most commonly is that of rhubarb root. But, others include senna, cascara as well as aloe. Consuming just a small amount of these elements through extras or a supplemental pill form will aid in the relief of constipation.

Movement Therapy

Another helpful alternative therapy for IBS is that of movement therapy. In this type of therapy, individuals have the ability to use their body to gain relaxation and help in dealing with the symptoms of IBS. Some of the best to consider include yoga and tai chi. Most individuals can benefit from adding one or both of these to their daily or every other day routine.

Doing yoga or tai chi can be helpful in several ways. The movements of the body can help to relive conditions such as pain in the abdomen, bloating, gas and diarrhea. There have been a few studies done to show this, most with benefits on a small scale being seen.

But, doing movement therapy has its benefits in other regards as well. For example, yoga can be beneficial not only to IBS but to improving the body's overall health and helping with maintaining the right weight.

As we discussed in earlier chapters, stress reduction is one of the most important things for you to take into consideration. When it comes to using movement therapy to treat IBS, you will be tackling the stress end of it. With these types of improvements, you can see benefits across the board in your health.

To add yoga or tai chi to your lifestyle, visit a local recreational center or gym. Sign up for a beginner's course. Doing this allows you to learn the true forms of these therapies and will give you the best possible response. Daily yoga is recommended, but any amount of it per week will show some benefits for you.

Mind Body Therapy

As we discussed early in this book, there is a connection to your emotional state and the IBS symptoms that you are experiencing. With the help of mind body therapies, you can actually improve your overall well being and reduce the amount and severity of symptoms of IBS.

Meditation is one of those types of activities. Meditation allows your body to relax and allows your mind to be put at ease. These things are imperative when it comes to fighting IBS. In addition, daily meditation allows for stress relief which can aid in the reduction of IBS symptoms itself.

Another type of mind body therapy that has proven to be quite beneficial is that of hypnotherapy. Even in some clinical trials, hypnotherapy has shown to be a tool to aid in the reduction of IBS symptoms. For it to be beneficial, you'll need to visit and have a hypnosis session each week. You will want to do this over several months for the best results.

During the hypnosis, the individual will have progressive relaxation done. This uses soothing images as well as sensations to help the individual's symptoms.

With effective hypnosis, there are several benefits that can be seen including pain in the abdomen being relieved, constipation that is reduced as is bloating and an overall improvement in quality of life.

To use hypnotherapy in your treatment for irritable bowel syndrome, find a qualified and experienced therapist. The largest challenge in making hypnosis work for you will be finding a therapist that is skilled at treatment of your condition.

In addition, it can be a costly alternative to other methods of treatment of IBS. Nevertheless, both of these mind body treatments can be quite beneficial.

Acupuncture

For thousands of years, acupuncture has been used to help in healing all types of medical conditions. There is no doubt that you will find some benefits in this ancient Chinese medicine. Today, it is widely used around the world and is growing in popularity.

What is acupuncture? For those that do not know, it seems like something out of a strange wizard's book, but in truth it is fairly simple to understand.

It works on the theory that there are channels of energy called meridians. Energy is called Qi. These channels course through the entire body. On these meridians there are three-hundred and sixty different acupuncture points. When you are healthy, the energy flows through the body easily through the channels. When you are ill, the energy flow is somehow disrupted. This is what causes symptoms like those that you face with IBS.

Acupuncture is then used at specific locations around your body to help release energy and then bring back the flow of the energy throughout the body.

What can acupuncture do for IBS then? There are several things that it can help with. Some individuals find relief from pain in the abdomen. Nausea and bloating can also be relieved through acupuncture.

If you would like to gain these benefits through acupuncture, your first goal will be to find an experienced and skilled acupuncturist. These individuals should have a good track record with helping individuals suffering specifically from irritable bowel syndrome.

Often times, acupuncture is made even better when it is paired with the correct ancient Chinese herbal remedies that have been used for centuries.

Acupuncture is a safe route to take when you use someone that is educated as well as experienced. Insuring this will insure a good result.

Probiotics

Probiotics can be helpful in treating IBS as well. They work by altering the intestinal flora. Probiotics are organisms that can help to regulate the bacteria within the intestines. By balancing these bacteria's, you will find benefit in the relief of the symptoms.

In your intestines there are intestinal flora, which are good bacteria. It is used to keep the GI tract working correctly. In addition, intestinal flora, which are actually organisms that that are throughout your intestines, also help with keeping your immune system healthy and providing for the secretion of fluids.

The thought is that perhaps the natural bacterial benefits can be used to help treat IBS as well. For this reason, probiotics have been used to simulate the intestinal flora. In some studies, probiotics have been beneficial in reducing the amount of pain that an individual experiences in the abdomen. The reduction of gas is also evident with the use of probiotics. For some individuals benefits have been seen in the function of the bowel with the help of probiotics too.

You can purchase probiotics readily in health food stores both online and in your local area. It is widely thought that they could be potentially beneficial to those that suffer from IBS, but there is much study need to provide this for sure.

Are Complimentary Therapies for You?

The end result of all of these different options is up to you. For some individuals, sticking with just the traditional medications is the only way to go. For others, the biggest benefit will come from the ability to avoid the use of medications that usually have harmful side effects. Yet, the bottom line is that it is a choice you need to make.

Remember that many of these complimentary therapies can be used in conjunction with the medications and lifestyle changes that your doctor has recommended. If you are unsure of how an herbal remedy will work with the medications that you are currently taking, ask your doctor about it first.

It is essential to find any and all relief that you can get from IBS symptoms. Complimentary therapies can be just the right choice.

Chapter 8: Irritable Bowel Syndrome Prevention

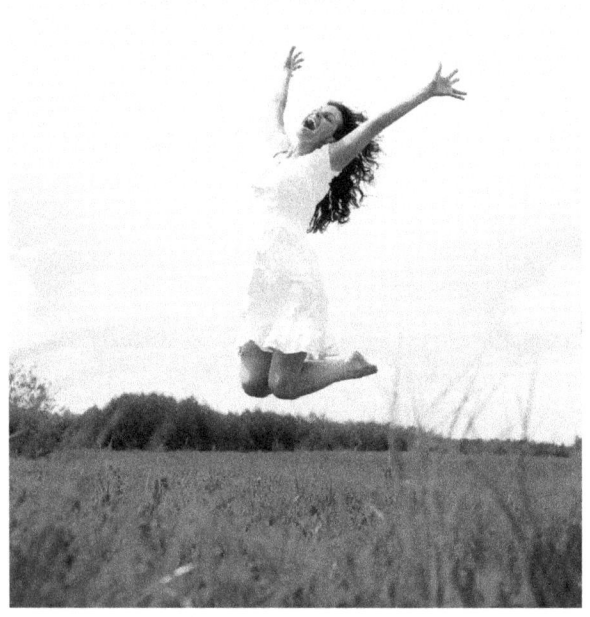

Prevention is the best medicine when it comes to irritable bowel syndrome. We can't stress that enough.

IBS is nothing to worry about when it happens. It is something to think about and plan for before the symptoms set in. Because we don't know what causes IBS in the first place, it is even more important for each of those that suffer from it to do what they can to stop it from happening in the first place.

Prevention is the best tool to make that happen. There are several things that you need to keep in mind when it comes to preventing the onset of irritable bowel syndrome symptoms.

In many ways, it is up to you and how you react to your condition that will determine just how severe and how often your symptoms arise. We can't cure irritable bowel syndrome yet, but there are things that we can do to prevent the symptoms from coming on.

Here are some of the best tools available to you to fight IBS through prevention.

Your Diet: Improving your diet is one of the best steps you can take to improving the quality of life you experience. There are plenty of opportunities for you to do this. Take our advice and get a food diary started. Find out just what is causing the most pronounced IBS symptoms for you and avoid those foods. While elimination diets can be helpful, you will also find that an overall well balanced diet can also be helpful in relieving IBS symptoms.

You should also consume the right amount of fiber for your needs. Those that face constipation are the most likely to need an additional source of fiber including with the help of supplements.

Counseling: There is no doubt about it, you need to work with your doctor to plan out the treatment that is right for you but you also should consider counseling. When it comes to IBS, it is essential to meet the emotional needs as well as the physical. In that, you want to consider talking to a psychologist or a psychiatrist.

By investing in a few sessions with a skilled psychologist, you will be better capable of reducing the levels of stress that can bring on IBS symptoms quickly. They will not only help you to reduce stress but also to help you to handle the events in your life that bring it on. They will teach you how to handle and relieve stress in such a way as to relieve your IBS symptoms.

Get Your Exercise: There is a need for your body to have physical movement. You need to get in physical movement and exercise daily. This can include such things as yoga, regular walking, aerobics, or other forms of physical activity.

Adding in the physical exercise keeps your body healthy as well as helps to alleviate the amount of stress you are under. It is easy to get in a walk here or there, or to sign up for yoga classes before or after work each day. By doing these things it can help you to stop the symptoms of IBS before they even start to happen.

Mind Therapy: While we mentioned getting counseling, there is a lot that you can do on your own to help reduce or prevent IBS symptoms when it comes to your mind. Meditation is a great tool for this. Make the time to allow yourself to clear your mind. It will help to relieve your stress and give you time to relax.

A great way to do this is to just come home and take a relaxing bath. Or find time before or after work when everyone is in bed to relax for a few minutes, alone with your thoughts.

Biofeedback: This is an excellent technique to learn in order to help you to reduce the amount of stress you are under. In this regard, you will learn how to accomplish this with the help of a machine. What it does is helps to reduce muscle tension and helps you to slow your heart rate. Although a machine will help you to do this at first, the goal is to show you how so that you can manage stress more effectively on your own.

Talk to your doctor about biofeedback opportunities. In most cases, they can be done in your local medical center or you can often find out more through your local hospital.

Hypnosis: As we mentioned earlier, the goal of hypnosis in regards of IBS is that of lowering the amount of pain that you are experiencing. With a skilled hypnotist, you can find benefits through relaxation for some or all of the symptoms you are facing due to IBS. It has been proven to be effective in reducing the amount of episodes of painful abdominal cramps as well as bloating.

In addition to helping with relaxation, a skilled hypnotist can actually help you to prevent the onset of severe symptoms by learning how to stop them when they begin to come on. For example, you will learn how to effectively relax your intestinal muscles by simply imaging them in a smooth and relaxed state.

Breathing: There is no doubt that the correct breathing techniques can also be quite helpful to those that face IBS. Learning to breathe correctly is going to be a big difference maker. Right now, as you are reading this, you are probably breathing from your chest. But, you can control your stress levels and relax easier if you learn to breathe from your diaphragm instead.

What does this have to do with IBS? Sit up straight and breathe so that your stomach expands. When you breathe out, you will naturally have your stomach muscles relaxing. During this relaxation, you will find that you allow your muscles of your abdomen to also relax, which in turn reduces the strain and pain being brought on by IBS.

Prevention is your goal when fighting IBS. Even if you can't manage to get in all of these various techniques to help you to find the relaxation and stress relief that you need, put aside just ten to twenty minutes per day for doing something that is relaxing. No matter what it is that makes you relax, do it. This in itself will help you to feel better and reduce the frequency of IBS symptoms.

Doing just one or two of these preventative measures will make the ultimate difference in your well being and health.

CHAPTER 9: CONCLUSION - MANAGING AND PREVENTING IRRITABLE BOWEL SYNDROME

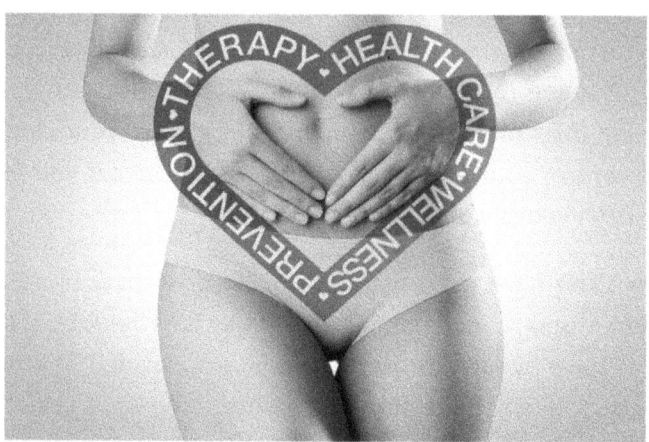

Irritable bowel syndrome is a condition which is likely to be something you face for many years to come. But, with a few effective tools and methods, you can manage your IBS in a way that lessens the frequency and the severity of your symptoms.

Here's your to do list to make this happen.

1. Manage your diet. Determine what foods could be worsening your symptoms, remove them or limit them from your diet. Get your fiber. Don't eat too much in one sitting.
2. Find out if your severe IBS warrants medication. Work with your doctor to find the right over the counter and prescription medications.
3. Relieve stress. Prevention is the best medicine to relieve stress. Use any of the methods that we've provided to help you to learn how to manage stress more effectively.

4. Consider and use alternative treatments for irritable bowel syndrome as we've discussed. One or more of these complimentary treatments can be quite effective.
5. Keep yourself educated and managing your own health. Keep up on the newest studies and the latest treatments for IBS. Manage your own healthcare by handling your symptoms through a whole body treatment.

Preventing IBS symptoms is not impossible, it is a challenge. Your best bet is to start with step one and work through all of them. Don't try to implement a lot of change at once either. Instead, work on improving your health by simply changing one thing at a time. Soon, you'll find that irritable bowel syndrome is something you can conquer.

MEET THE AUTHOR

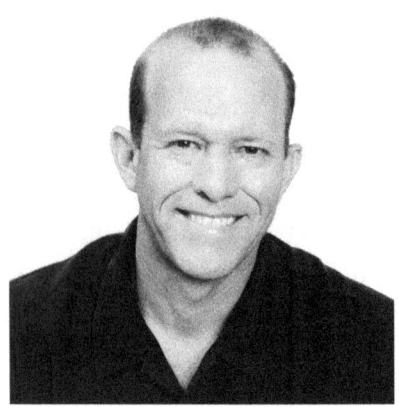

Hayden Anderson has a passion for helping others obtain peace and wellness. Sometimes that means changing lifestyle habits and addressing medical complexities through nutrition and alternative medicine. Hayden has years of experience in the area of holistic health, yoga, and meditation. He uses his experience and knowledge to change people's perception of eastern medicine.

As a kid Hayden suffered from a chronic illness that doctor's treated with medication. Hayden's parents were satisfied with doctor's maintaining his condition but Hayden wanted more. At nineteen Hayden became obsessed with eastern medicine and took control of his health. Through the use of herbs and dietary changes to complement his blood type, he was able throw away prescription medication that he had taken daily for as long as he could remember. He never looked back and is passionate about sharing his knowledge with others.

Hayden, his wife and kids enjoy spending time outdoors, growing their own food and herbs, sharing their day with each other around the family dinner table and game nights with old fashioned board games like Parcheesi, Aggravation, Sorry, Clue and Life.